Heart Murmurs Made Easy

A Practical Guide for Medical and Nursing Students

Dr. Sivajith P R

Respect copyright
Say no to piracy

Copyright © 2024-25 Dr. SIVAJITH PR

Heart Murmurs Made Easy - 1st edition

All rights reserved. No part of this book may be reproduced, stored in a retrieval system, or transmitted in any form or by any means, electronic, mechanical, photocopying, recording, or otherwise, without the express written permission of the author.

Message from the author

This book is intended for medical & nursing students seeking to enhance their understanding of cardiac murmurs in a clear and effective manner.

Prior to delving into this text, readers should possess a foundational knowledge of cardiac anatomy (including valves and major cardiac vessels), heart development (with a focus on the interventricular and interatrial septum), the cardiac cycle, and auscultation. This background knowledge will facilitate a deeper comprehension of the concepts discussed within.

The realm of cardiac murmurs is vast, encompassing numerous mechanisms and cardiodynamic principles. In this book, I have distilled the most essential concepts that every clinical practitioner should be familiar with in order to accurately auscultate and interpret murmurs. Complex topics have been omitted to maintain simplicity and clarity.

Included within these pages are practical clinical tips and strategies for distinguishing between murmurs of different etiologies. Additionally, a basic overview of congenital cardiac diseases, a crucial topic in pediatrics, is provided.

I trust that you will find this book both enjoyable and beneficial to your academic and professional pursuits. Your feedback and suggestions are welcomed at sivajithpr93@gmail.com.

Wishing you a fruitful learning experience.

Table of contents

1. Auscultatory areas
2. Heart sounds
3. Classification of murmurs
4. How to describe a murmur
5. Clinical approach to murmur
6. Valvular heart diseases

   - Aortic valve diseases
   - Mitral valve diseases
   - Tricuspid valve diseases
   - Pulmonary valve diseases

7. Congenital heart diseases

   - Ventricular septal defect
   - Atrial septal defect
   - Patent ductus arteriosus
   - Tetralogy of fallot

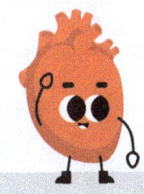

Auscultatory Areas

- Auscultatory areas are the places on the chest wall where we place our stethoscope to hear heart sounds and murmurs.

- There are mainly 5 auscultatory areas, namely:
    1. Mitral area
    2. Tricuspid area
    3. Pulmonary area
    4. Aortic area
    5. Erb's point/area

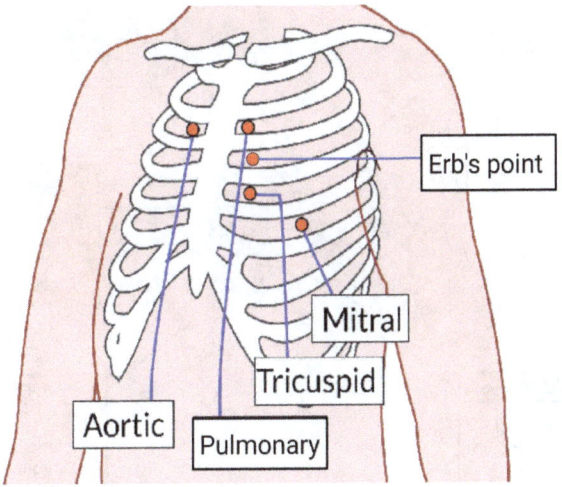

Img[1]: Auscultatory areas (adapted from the work of Theodore-Dimitriou)

Area	Location
Mitral area	Corresponds to apex beat
Tricuspid area	Left 4th ICS adjacent to the sternal border
Erb's area	Left 3rd ICS adjacent to the sternal border
Aortic area	Right 2nd ICS adjacent to the sternal border
Pulmonary area	Left 2nd ICS adjacent to the sternal border

**ICS - Intercostal space

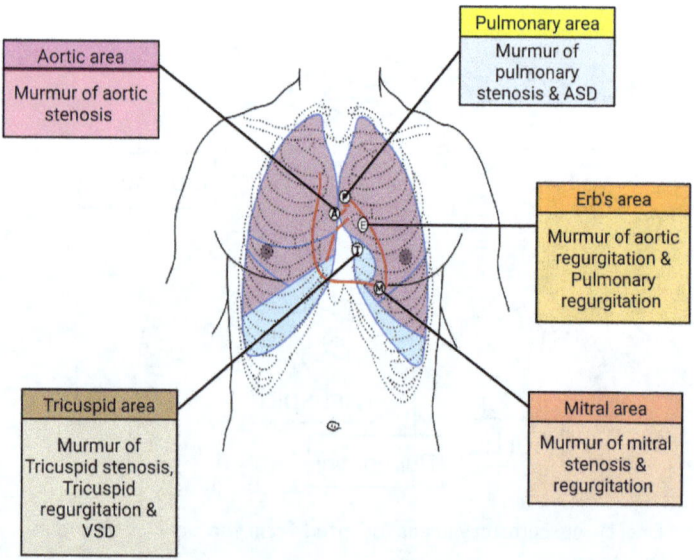

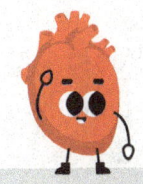

Heart Sounds

Normal Heart Sounds

The normal heart sounds include S1 and S2.

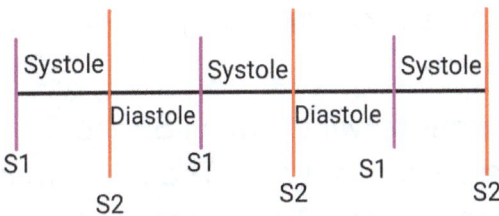

S1 (First heart sound)

- S1 (first heart sound) is produced as a result of the closure of the mitral and tricuspid valves.
- It can be heard over all the auscultatory areas but is best heard at the mitral area/apex.
- It synchronizes with carotid pulsation.

S2 (second heart sound)

- S2 (second heart sound) is produced as a result of the closure of the aortic and pulmonary valves.

- Although these two valves close almost simultaneously, the pulmonic valve usually lags slightly behind. Therefore, under certain circumstances, the two components of the second sound (aortic component [A2] & Pulmonary component [P2]) may be heard separately. This is called the splitting of the second heart sound.
- Splitting is accentuated by the process of inspiration.
- The time interval between S1 and S2 corresponds to systole. The time interval between S2 and S1 corresponds to diastole.

Gallop rhythms

Gallop rhythms include S3 (Third heart sound) and S4 (Fourth heart sound). They are abnormal and heard in pathological conditions like heart failure, hypertension, etc.

S3 (Third heart sound)

- S3 is produced as a result of ventricular filling.
- It is usually pathological.

- It is heard immediately following S2.
- Heard in heart failure, mitral regurgitation, and tricuspid regurgitation.

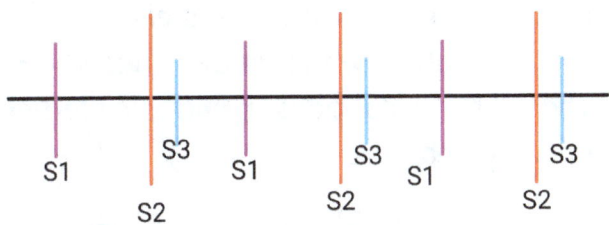

S4 (Fourth heart sound)

- S4 is produced as a result of forcible atrial contraction (to fill non-compliant ventricles in ventricular hypertrophy or infarct).
- It is heard immediately preceding S1.
- Heard in systemic hypertension, aortic-stenosis, pulmonary hypertension, pulmonary stenosis, and myocardial infarction.

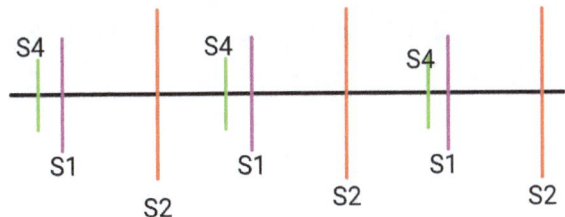

Clicks and Snaps

- Opening snap: Blood flow through a stenosed mitral valve gives rise to a high-pitched sound, which is best heard along the left sternal border and is called an opening snap.

- Ejection click: Blood flow through a stenosed aortic valve gives rise to a short, high-pitched sound immediately after S1, which is called an ejection click.

Murmurs

Murmurs are the abnormal sounds produced as a result turbulent flow of the blood.

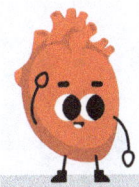

Classification of Heart Murmurs

Murmurs are the abnormal sounds produced as a result of turbulent blood flow. The causes of the turbulence may be:

1. A narrowed (stenosed) valve.
2. A malfunctioning valve that allows regurgitant blood flow.
3. A congenital defect of the ventricular or atrial wall.
4. Cardiomyopathies.
5. A defect between the aorta and the pulmonary artery (e.g., Patent ductus arteriosus).
6. An increased flow of blood (e.g., with fever, anemia, pregnancy, hyperthyroidism, etc).

Murmurs can be broadly classified into systolic murmurs, diastolic murmurs, and continuous murmurs.

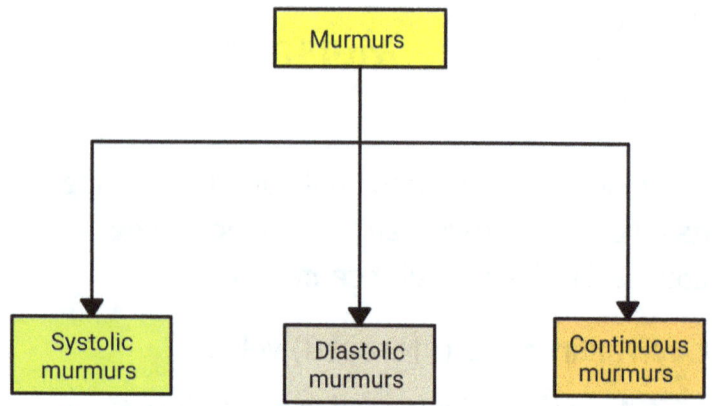

Timing to systole or diastole is achieved by palpation of the carotid pulse while auscultating. A systolic murmur occurs at the same time as the carotid pulse, whereas a diastolic murmur occurs in the pause between carotid pulses.

Systolic murmurs

They are the murmurs which are produced during the systolic phase of the cardiac cycle. It can be further divided into :

Early systolic murmur

Occurs during the early stages of systole. It is heard in mitral regurgitation, ventricular septal defect, and tricuspid regurgitation.

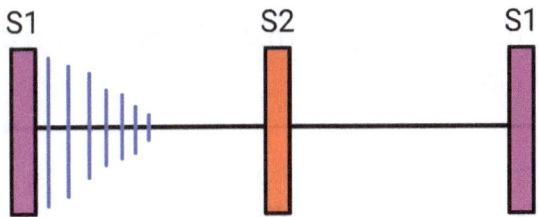

Ejection systolic murmur (Midsystolic murmur)

Occurs during midsystole. It is a crescendo-decrescendo murmur or saw-shaped murmur. Heard in aortic stenosis and pulmonary stenosis.

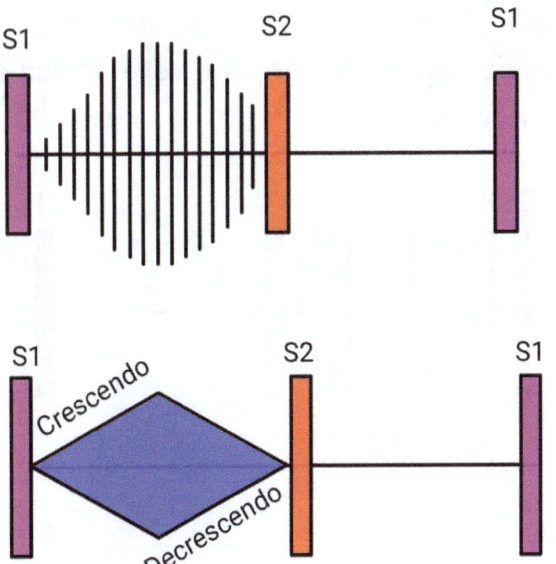

Late systolic murmur

Occurs during late systole. Heard in mitral valve prolapse.

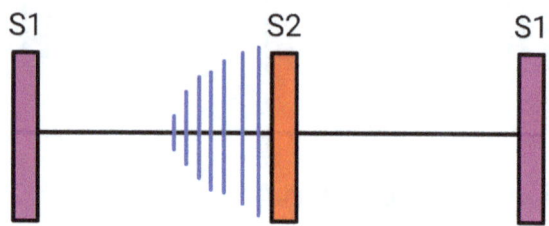

Pansystolic murmur

Extends throughout the systole. Here S1 and S2 cannot be heard separately from the murmur. Heard in Mitral regurgitation, Tricuspid regurgitation, and ventricular septal defect (VSD).

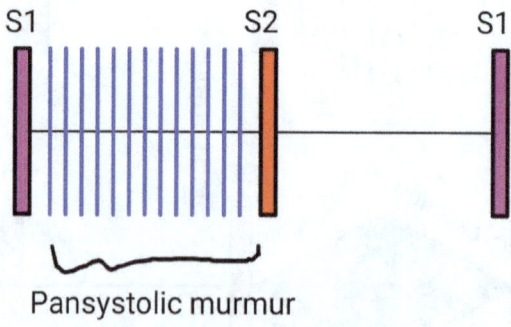

Pansystolic murmur

Diastolic murmurs

Diastolic murmurs can be Early diastolic, Mid diastolic and late diastolic.

Early diastolic murmur
Early diastolic murmur is heard in aortic regurgitation and pulmonic regurgitation.

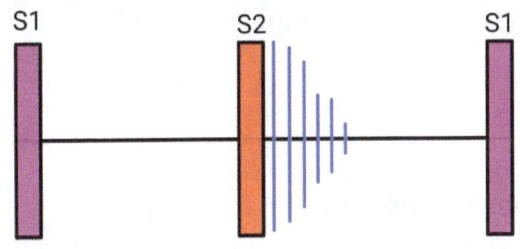

Mid-diastolic murmur
Mid-diastolic murmur is heard in mitral stenosis and tricuspid stenosis.

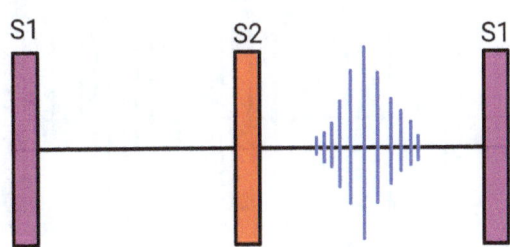

Late diastolic murmur

Late-diastolic murmur is heard in mitral stenosis, tricuspid stenosis, myxoma and complete heart block (3rd degree).

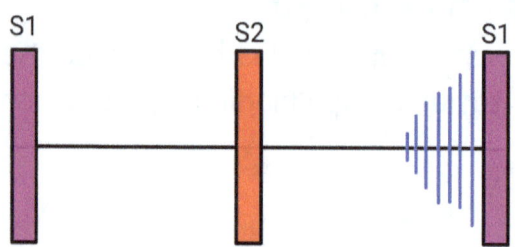

Continous murmurs

Continuous murmurs are heard continuously during both systole and diastole. They are heard in patent ductus arteriosus, shunts, and coarctation of the aorta.

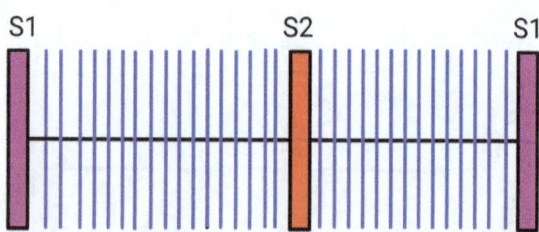

Other types of murmurs

Innocent murmurs

Seen in children. It is mostly found in the early age group and then slowly disappears as the children start to grow. It is not associated with any structural heart disease and is quite benign.

Characteristics of an Innocent murmur are :

1. Best heard over the Pulmonary area and localized.
2. Systolic in nature.
3. Normally grade II murmur, which is soft and no thrill present.
4. Best heard in the supine position and disappears in the upright position. Sometimes the murmur is heard after exercise or crying.
5. S1 and S2 are heard normally.
6. Symptomless.
7. ECG, ECHO, and Chest X-ray normal.

Functional murmurs

This occurs due to increased blood flow as a result of some cardiac pathologies. E.g.:

- Early diastolic Graham Steell murmur in pulmonary hypertension.
- Austin Flint murmur (due to functional MS) in aortic regurgitation.

Flow murmurs

It is not pathological. It occurs as a result of increased blood flow as seen in severe anemia, thyrotoxicosis, fever... etc.

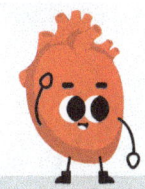

How to Describe Murmurs

Murmurs are due to turbulence of blood at or near a valve or an abnormal communication within or outside the heart. Once we have identified the presence of the murmur, we should describe it under the following headings:

1. Timing of murmur (Whether it is systolic, diastolic, or continuous)
2. Area of maximum intensity
3. Frequency or pitch
4. Intensity of murmur
5. Conduction & transmission of murmur
6. Postural variation
7. Variation with respiration

1. Timing & duration of murmur

Based on timing and duration, murmurs are classified into:

- Systolic murmur (heard between S1 and S2)

1. Ejection systolic
2. Pansystolic
3. Early systolic
4. Late systolic

- Diastolic murmur (heard between S2 & S1)

  1. Early diastolic
  2. Mid diastolic
  3. Late diastolic

- Continuous murmur (heard both during systole and diastole without any relation to the heart sounds)

Describe whether the murmur is systolic, diastolic, or continuous (e.g., A pansystolic murmur is heard at the mitral area)

2. Area of maximum intensity

Describe the area where the murmur is maximally heard (Eg: A pansystolic murmur is heard, which is best appreciated at the mitral area.)

3. Frequency or pitch

- Murmurs can be low, medium, or high-pitched. Usually, the high-pitched murmurs are soft and blowing in character, whereas low-pitched murmurs are rough, and some of them are rumbling.
- Low-pitch murmurs are better heard with the bell of the stethoscope.
- High-pitch murmurs are better heard with the diaphragm of the stethoscope.

4. Intensity of murmur

Based on the intensity, murmur is graded as follows (Levine and Freeman's grading):

- Grade 1: Murmur, which is not heard immediately on auscultation, requires a quiet surrounding and an experienced listener, and repeated auscultation.
- Grade 2: A soft murmur immediately audible in quiet surroundings.
- Grade 3: A prominent murmur.
- Grade 4: A loud murmur with a thrill.
- Grade 5: A still louder murmur can be heard with the edge of the stethoscope touching the chest.

- Grade 6: A murmur audible with the stethoscope held off the chest or without the stethoscope.

5. Conduction & radiation

- Conduction means the selective propagation of a murmur along a line so that it is heard with the same or sometimes greater intensity.
- Transmission or radiation means that the murmur is heard with lesser intensity away from the original site.

6. Variation with Posture and Respiration

- If the murmur is better heard in a sitting and leaning forward position with breath held in expiration, then it would be the murmur of aortic valve abnormalities (AR or AS).
- If a murmur is better heard in the left lateral position with breath held in expiration, then it would be the murmur of mitral valve abnormalities (MR or MS).

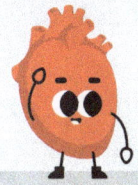

Clinical Approach to Heart Murmurs

Once we have identified the presence of the murmur, we should follow the following steps for a systematic analysis and interpretation.

Step 1 : Auscultation

During auscultation, determine the following:

1) The auscultatory area on which the murmur can be heard most clearly and loudly.

For example:

- Murmurs of mitral valve abnormalities are better heard at the mitral area.
- Murmurs of aortic valve abnormalities are better heard at the aortic area.
- Murmurs of pulmonary valves are better heard at the pulmonary area.
- Murmurs of tricuspid valves are better heard at the tricuspid area.

2) Whether it is better heard with the diaphragm of the stethoscope or the bell of the stethoscope.

- Better heard with bell: low-pitch murmurs.
- Better heard with diaphragm: high-pitch murmurs.

3) Postural variation and relation with respiration.

- If the murmur is better heard in a sitting and leaning forward position with breath held in expiration, then it would be the murmur of aortic valve abnormalities (AR or AS).
- If a murmur is better heard in the left lateral position with breath held in expiration, then it would be the murmur of mitral valve abnormalities (MR or MS).

4) Assess the intensity of the murmur and grade it.

Grade 1 : Very faint murmur
Grade 2 : Faint murmur
Grade 3 : Loudest murmur without thrill
Grade 4 : Murmur with thrill
Grade 5 : Loud murmur with thrill
Grade 6 : Loudest murmur with thrill

** A palpable murmur is called "Thrill"

5) Radiation of murmur

In some cases, a murmur may conduct/radiate to areas other than auscultatory areas. For example:
- Murmur of aortic stenosis radiates to the carotids bilaterally.
- Murmur of mitral regurgitation radiates to the axilla.

Step 2: Determine the type

Determine whether the murmur is systolic or diastolic.

- A murmur that coincides with carotid pulsation is considered a systolic murmur.
- A murmur that does not coincide with carotid pulsation is considered a diastolic murmur

Step 3: Assessment of apex beat

Assessment of the apex beat will be useful in arriving at a clinical diagnosis.

Types of apex	Characterstic features
Normal apex beat	* Position : 5th ICS * Confined to one ICS * Character: palpating finger is lifted, but not above the plane of adjoining ribs
Forcible apex beat	* Position : 6th, 7th or 8th ICS * Confined to more than one ICS * Character: palpating finger is lifted above the plane of adjoining ribs but is ill-sustained * Seen in AR & MR
Heaving apex beat	* Position : 5th ICS * Confined to one ICS * Character: palpating finger is lifted above the plane of adjoining ribs and is sustained * Seen in AS
Tapping apex beat	* Position : 5th ICS * Confined to one ICS * Character: palpating finger is not lifted but S1 is felt as a definitive tap * Seen in MS

Step 4: Correlation with history

- Correlate the clinical diagnosis with the patient's history and symptoms.
- In history, always ask about the history of rheumatic fever.

Step 5: Investigations

- Echocardiography (ECHO) is the gold standard investigation.
- X-ray may show cardiomegaly.

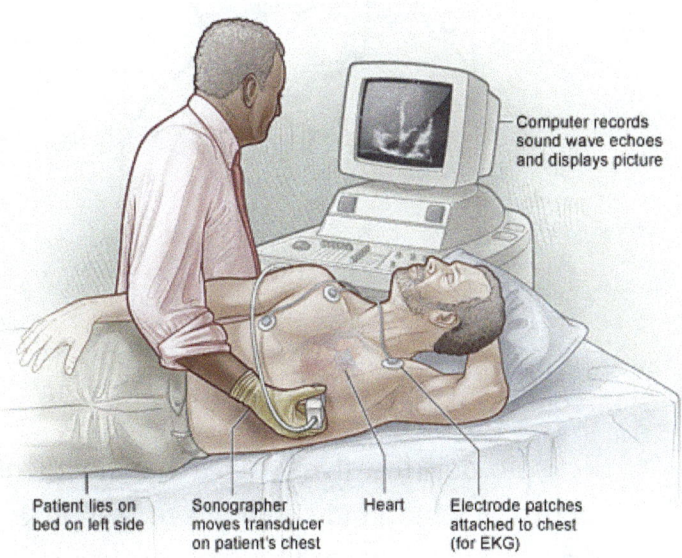

Img: Echocardiography

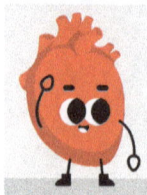

Aortic Valve Diseases

Includes Aortic stenosis & Aortic regurgitation.

Aortic stenosis

It is the narrowing of the aortic valve opening.

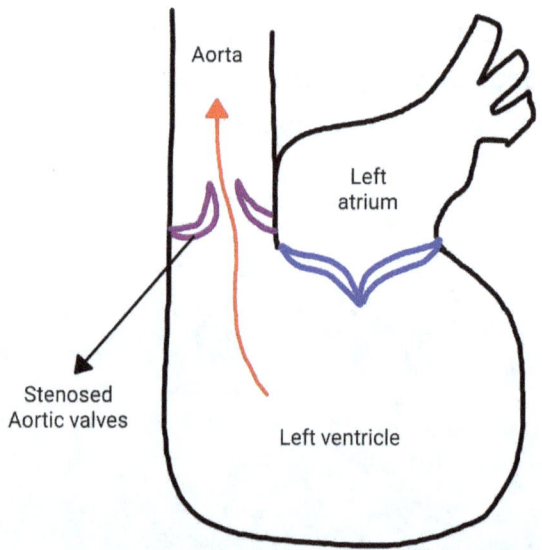

Major causes of aortic stenosis are:

- Bicuspid aortic valves - It is a congenital condition which may also present in late life.
- Rheumatic heart disease.

- Age-related calcific degeneration of the aortic valve.

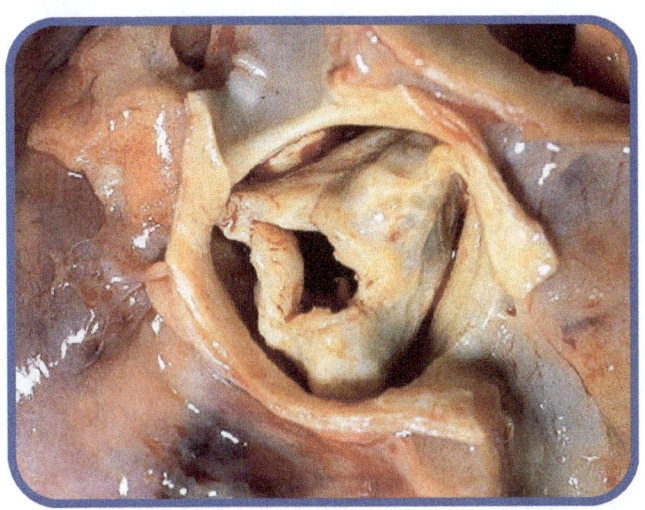

Autopsy specimen of a patient with rheumatic heart disease showing a thickened and calcified aortic valve.

Symptoms of aortic stenosis are; (Mnemonic: SAD)

1. Exertional Syncope
2. Exertional Angina
3. Exertional Dyspnoea

Signs of aortic stenosis are;

- Pulse: Low volume slow rising pulse (pulsus parvus et tardus)

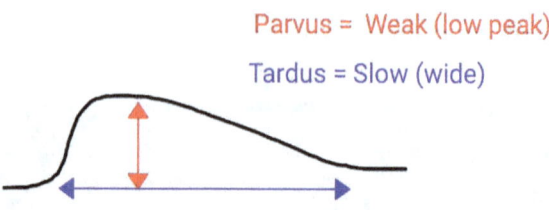

Img: pulsus parvus et tardus

- Apex beat will be heaving type, i.e., palpating fingers will be raised above the plane of adjoining ribs and it is sustained. Apex beat will be palpable at 5th ICS, 1cm lateral to the mid-clavicular line and limited to one ICS.

- On auscultation, an ejection systolic murmur could be heard at the aortic area, which radiates bilaterally to the carotids. It is best heard with the patient sitting and leaning forward with breath held in expiration.

- An ejection click may be present (it is heard just after S1 because of the sudden opening of aortic and pulmonary valves).

- Occasionally, the murmur of Aortic stenosis may be transmitted to the mitral area and is known as Gallavardin's phenomenon.

- S2 is muffled/soft.

- The murmur of AS is a crescendo-decrescendo murmur or saw-like murmur as shown in the diagram.

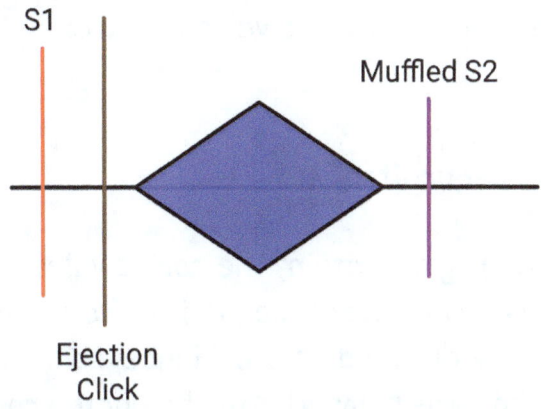

Investigations

- X-ray chest: Normal-sized heart due to concentric left ventricular hypertrophy (In concentric hypertrophy, ventricular muscle mass increases but volume remains the same).

- ECG: Shows features of left ventricular hypertrophy.
- Echocardiography: It is the investigation of choice.

Management

- Management of LVH, angina atrial fibrillation
- In young patients: Valvotomy can be done.
- In adults and elders: Valvuloplasty.
- Calcific AS: Aortic valve replacement.

Aortic regurgitation

In aortic regurgitation, the aortic valve becomes incompetent, i.e., it fails to close completely during diastole. Hence, some of the blood that was pumped into the aorta from the left ventricle during systole regurgitates back into the left ventricle during diastole. As a result of this, the left ventricle has to work hard to pump out excessive blood, leading to eccentric hypertrophy of the left ventricle and eventually its failure.

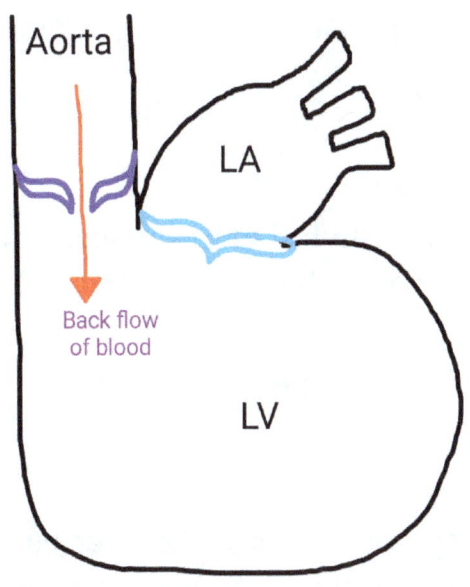

Causes of Aortic regurgitation

Congenital causes: Bicuspid aortic valve

Acquired causes:
- Rheumatic heart disease
- Trauma
- Infective endocarditis
- Conditions causing aortic root dilatation such as Marfan's syndrome, aortic aneurysm, syphilis... Etc

Symptoms of Aortic regurgitation

- Dyspnoea
- Angina
- Palpitations
- Features of LVF (Left ventricular failure) or CCF (Congestive cardiac failure)

Signs of Aortic regurgitation

Pulse:

Collapsing pulse or water hammer pulse. It is characterized by an abrupt upstroke and downstroke with an ill-sustained plateau.

Normal pulse

Collapsing pulse
(Abrupt upstroke and downstroke.
No plateau)

Blood pressure:

High systolic and low diastolic BP, i.e., wide pulse pressure.

Apex beat:

Forcible apex beat, i.e.,

- Palpating finger is lifted above the plane of adjoining ribs but not sustained.
- Apex is shifted downward and outward (Felt at 6th, 7th, or 8th ICS) because of eccentric hypertrophy of the left ventricle).
- Felt in more than one ICS.

Peripheral signs of Aortic regurgitation

- Quincke's sign - Pulsation of nail beds.
- Corrigan's sign - Prominent carotid pulsations in the neck.
- Hill's sign - Increase in the femoral artery systolic BP > 20 mm Hg above the brachial artery systolic BP.
- Duroziez's murmur - Diastolic murmur on compression of the femoral artery distally.

- Traube's sign - Pistol shot sound produced on pressing the stethoscope over the femoral artery.
- De Musset's sign - To and fro head nodding synchronous with carotid pulsation.

On auscultation;

- S2 muffled.
- A soft blowing early diastolic murmur can be heard at the Aortic and Erb's areas. It is best heard with the patient sitting and leaning forward with breath held in expiration. The murmur may radiate towards the axilla and apex.

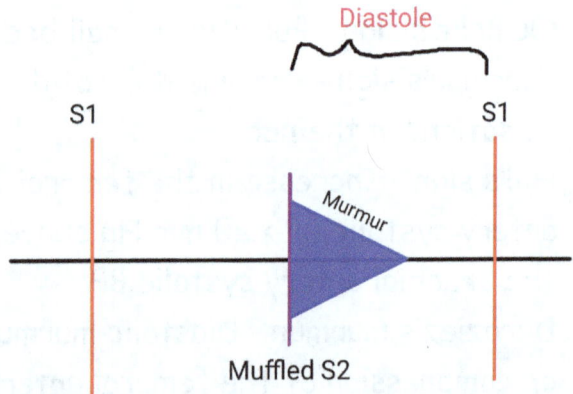

- Another murmur called Austin Flint murmur could be heard at the mitral area, which is a mid-diastolic rumbling murmur of functional mitral stenosis (because the regurgitant jet of blood strikes the mitral valve and stenoses it).

Investigations :

- Chest X-ray: shows Cardiomegaly (due to eccentric hypertrophy of the left ventricle), Dilatation of the aortic root, and Calcified aortic valve.
- ECG: Shows signs of LVH.
- Echocardiography is the investigation of choice.

Treatment :

- Management of cardiac failure.
- Treatment of underlying causes like syphilis or rheumatic heart disease.
- Aortic valve replacement.
- In some cases, aortic root replacement is also done along with valve replacement.

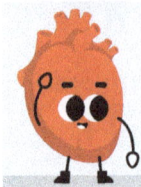

Murmur of HOCM

HOCM (Hypertrophic Obstructive Cardiomyopathy) is a type of Cardiomyopathy in which hypertrophy of the myocardium causes obstruction to the left ventricular outflow, which produces an ejection systolic murmur similar to aortic stenosis. The features that help to differentiate it from an aortic stenosis murmur are:

- It is best heard at the left sternal border.
- No radiation to the carotids.
- Intensity of the murmur decreases with the squatting position.

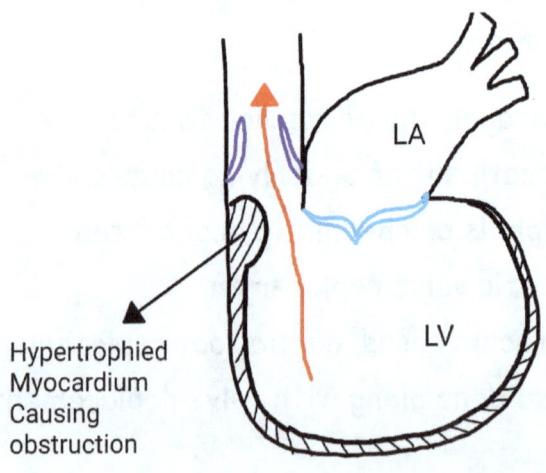

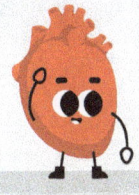

Mitral Valve Diseases

Mitral stenosis (MS)

- It is the narrowing of the mitral valve orifice.

- Rheumatic heart disease is the most common cause of mitral stenosis. In rheumatic heart disease, progressive fibrosis and calcification of valve leaflets occur, which results in narrowing of the mitral valve orifice. This gives the valve orifice a typical appearance of a fish mouth.

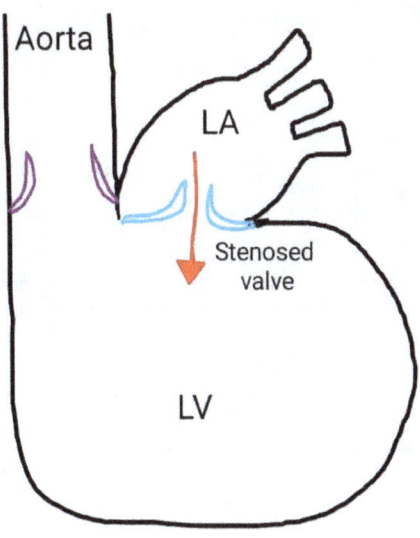

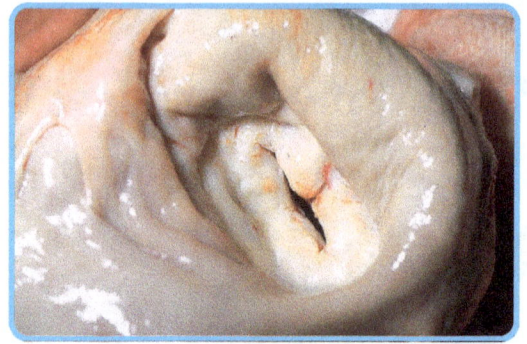

Autopsy specimen of a patient with rheumatic heart disease showing a typical fish-mouth appearance of stenosed mitral valve

Pathogenesis of MS

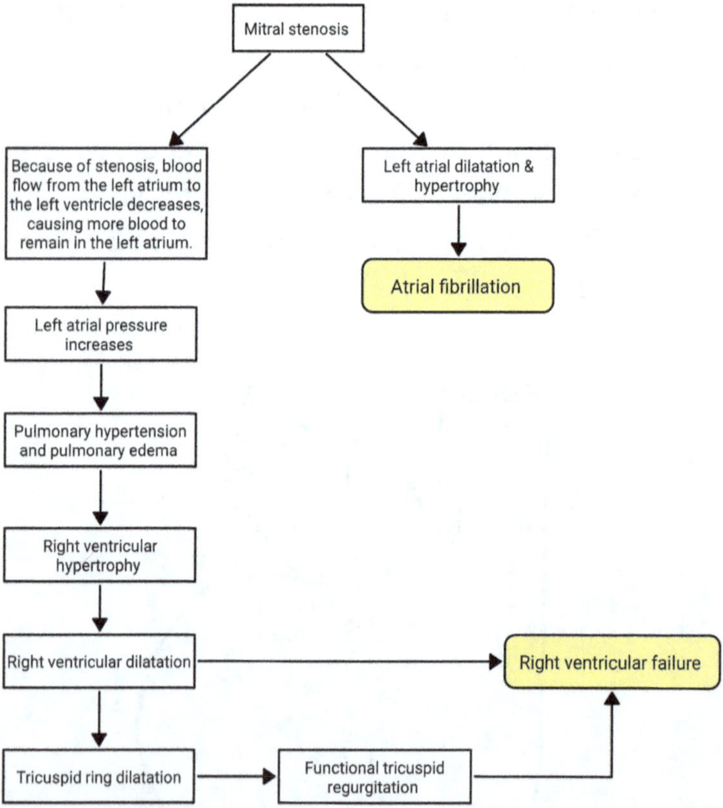

```
                        ┌──────────────────┐
                        │ Mitral stenosis  │
                        └──────────────────┘
                         /              \
                        /                \
┌──────────────────────────┐      ┌──────────────────────┐
│ Because of stenosis,     │      │ Left atrial          │
│ blood flow from the left │      │ dilatation &         │
│ atrium to the left       │      │ hypertrophy          │
│ ventricle decreases,     │      └──────────────────────┘
│ causing more blood to    │                │
│ remain in the left       │                ▼
│ atrium.                  │      ┌──────────────────────┐
└──────────────────────────┘      │ Atrial fibrillation  │
             │                    └──────────────────────┘
             ▼
┌──────────────────────┐
│ Left atrial pressure │
│ increases            │
└──────────────────────┘
             │
             ▼
┌──────────────────────┐
│ Pulmonary hypertension│
│ and pulmonary edema  │
└──────────────────────┘
             │
             ▼
┌──────────────────────┐
│ Right ventricular    │
│ hypertrophy          │
└──────────────────────┘
             │
             ▼
┌──────────────────────┐         ┌──────────────────────┐
│ Right ventricular    │────────▶│ Right ventricular    │
│ dilatation           │         │ failure              │
└──────────────────────┘         └──────────────────────┘
             │                              ▲
             ▼                              │
┌──────────────────────┐    ┌──────────────────────────┐
│ Tricuspid ring       │───▶│ Functional tricuspid     │
│ dilatation           │    │ regurgitation            │
└──────────────────────┘    └──────────────────────────┘
```

Symptoms

- Dyspnoea
- Cough with hemoptysis - Due to pulmonary edema
- Paroxysmal nocturnal dyspnea & Orthopnoea
- Features of atrial fibrillation
- Features of right heart failure (Edema, Tender hepatomegaly & Elevated JVP)

Signs

Mitral facies:

Pinkish-purple patches on the cheeks. It usually resembles malar rashes seen in SLE.

Pulse:

Irregularly irregular pulse if atrial fibrillation develops as a complication.

Apex beat:

Tapping in character and normal in position (left 5th intercostal space).

Left parasternal heave

Due to right ventricular hypertrophy.

On auscultation :

- Loud S1.
- A mid-diastolic rumbling murmur with presystolic accentuation can be heard at the mitral area, which is best heard when the patient is in the left lateral position with breath held in expiration.
- An opening snap can be heard just after S2.
- Loud P2 if there is pulmonary hypertension.

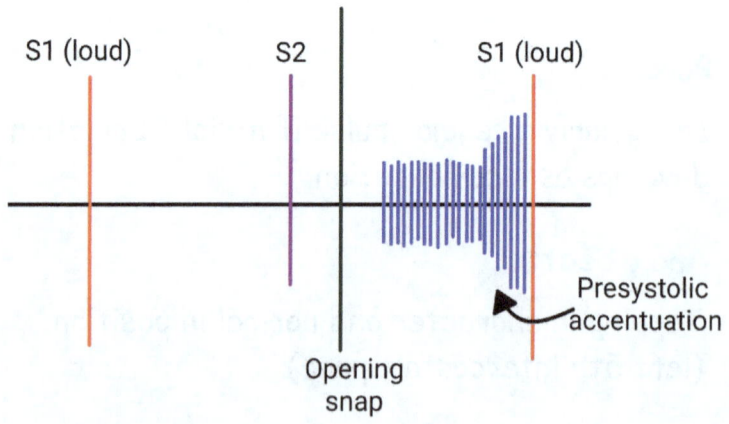

Img: Mid-diastolic murmur of MS

Complications of MS:

- Pulmonary-hypertension
- Right ventricular failure
- Atrial fibrillation
- Atrial flutter
- Embolism
- Hemoptysis
- Infective endocarditis

Investigations

- Chest X-ray: Right ventricular hypertrophy and features of pulmonary edema.
- ECG: Wide and notched (bifid) P wave due to left atrial hypertrophy (P Mitrale).
- Echocardiography is the investigation of choice.

Treatment

- Treatment of heart failure & atrial fibrillation
- Surgical interventions such as valvulotomy, valvuloplasty, or valve replacement
- Prophylaxis for rheumatic fever & infective endocarditis

Mitral regurgitation (MR)

In Mitral regurgitation, the mitral valves are incompetent, i.e., they fail to close completely and firmly. Hence, during ventricular systole (contraction), some blood regurgitates back from the left ventricle into the left atrium.

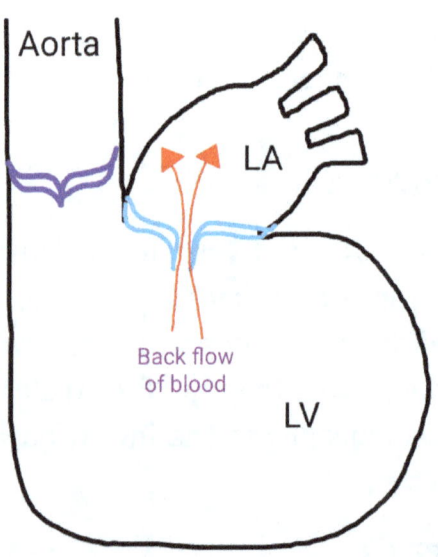

Causes of MR

1. Mitral Valve Prolapse (MVP)

- Mitral valve prolapse is also known as Barlow's syndrome or floppy valve syndrome.

- It is a condition in which part of one or both flaps of the mitral valve bulge (prolapse) upward into the left atrium.
- This is due to the myxomatous degeneration of valve leaflets.
- As a result of this, the valve leaflets fail to close smoothly or evenly, resulting in mitral regurgitation.

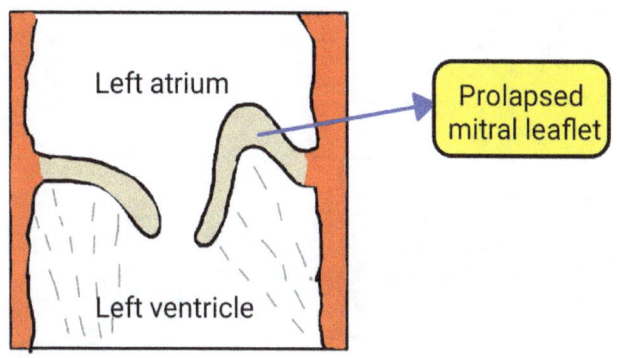

2. Rheumatic heart disease

3. Congenital anomalies

4. Myocardial infarction (Ischemic heart disease)

5. Infective endocarditis

Pathogenesis of MR

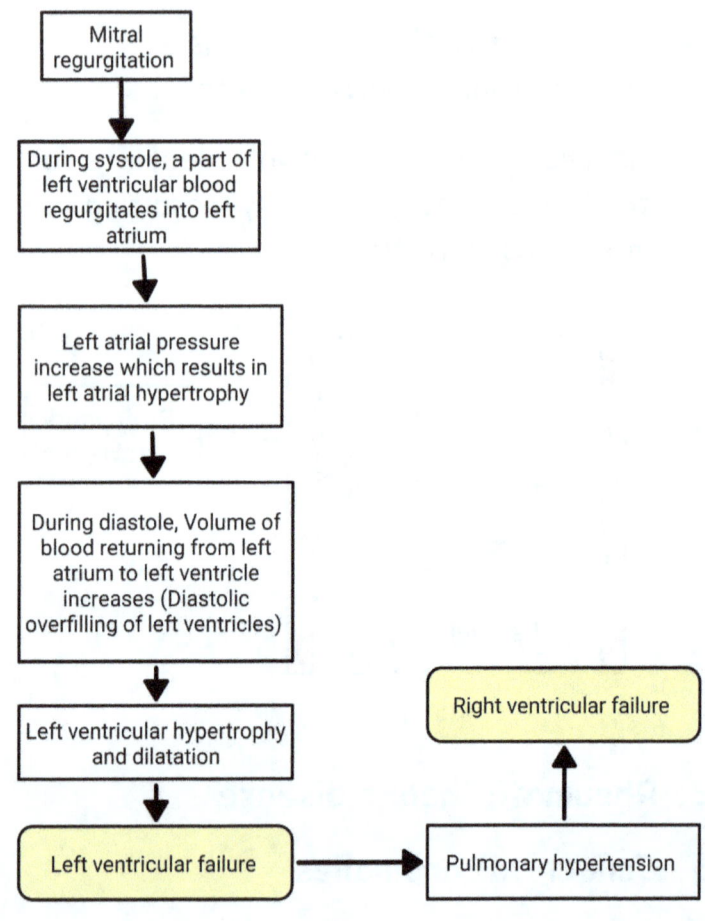

Symptoms of MR:

- Exertional dyspnea & fatigue
- Paroxysmal nocturnal dyspnea & orthopnea - due to left ventricular failure
- Features of right heart failure such as edema, ascites, elevated JVP, etc.
- Palpitations - due to atrial fibrillation

Signs of MR:

Pulse

Irregularly irregular pulse if atrial fibrillation present.

Apex beat

Forcible apex beat i.e.

- Palpating finger is lifted above the plane of adjoining ribs but not sustained.
- Apex is shifted downward and outward (Felt at 6th, 7th, or 8th ICS) because of eccentric hypertrophy of the left ventricle.
- Felt in more than one ICS.

Features of RVH

There will be features of right ventricular hypertrophy such as a left parasternal heave and epigastric pulsation.

On auscultation

- S1 soft
- A high-pitched pansystolic murmur can be heard at the mitral area, which is best heard with the patient in the left lateral position with breath held in expiration. The murmur is radiated towards the left axilla and inferior angle of the left scapula (hallmark of diagnosis)

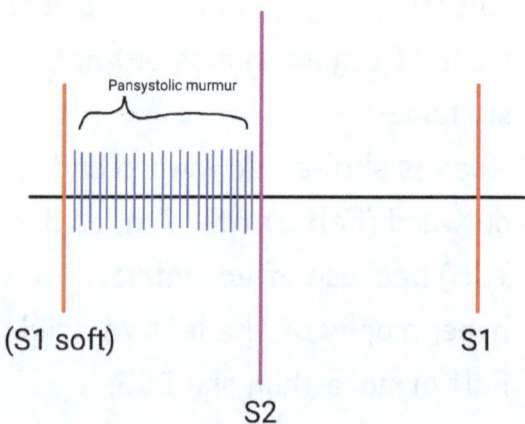

Signs of heart failure

If LVF is present,

- S3 is heard (called triple gallop rhythm - S1, S2, S3)
- Fine crepitations are heard at lung bases (pulmonary edema)
- Pulsus alternans

If RVF is present,

- Jugular venous pressure is raised
- Tender hepatomegaly is present
- Bipedal edema is seen

Complications

- Heart failure - Left heart failure, right heart failure, or congestive heart failure.
- Atrial fibrillation
- Infective endocarditis
- Recurrent respiratory infections

Investigations

- Chest X-ray: Hypertrophied left atrium, left ventricle & right ventricle
- ECG: Features of atrial fibrillation
- ECHO: Gold standard investigation

Management

- Treatment of heart failure
- Treatment of atrial fibrillation
- Mitral valve repair or replacement

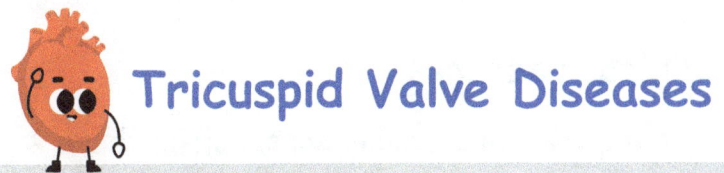

Tricuspid Valve Diseases

Tricuspid regurgitation (TR)

Tricuspid regurgitation is common, and mostly it occurs as a result of right ventricular dilation due to right heart failure or biventricular failure.

Causes:

Causes can be primary or secondary.

Primary causes

- Rheumatic heart disease
- Infective endocarditis
- Ebstein's anomaly

Secondary causes

- Right ventricular failure
- Biventricular failure (Congestive cardiac failure)
- Pulmonary hypertension

Clinical features

- Symptoms are usually nonspecific; there may be fatigue and breathlessness.
- There may be signs of right heart failure such as bilateral pedal edema, tender-hepatomegaly, ascites, and elevated JVP.
- On auscultation, a pansystolic murmur can be heard at the tricuspid area, which is best heard during inspiration.

Investigations

Echocardiography is the investigation of choice.

Management

Treat heart failure first. Tricuspid-regurgitation due to right ventricular dilation secondary to right heart failure will improve once heart failure is completely treated. If valves are damaged due to endocarditis, we can opt for valve repair. Those with rheumatic damage may require valve replacement.

Tricuspid stenosis (TS)

Usually rheumatic in origin and nearly always occur in association with mitral and aortic valve diseases.

Clinical features

- There may be features of right heart failure such as edema, ascites, elevated JVP, and hepatic discomfort.
- On auscultation, a mid-diastolic murmur can be heard at the mitral area, which is best heard with breath held in inspiration.

Investigations

Echocardiography is the investigation of choice

Management

- Valve replacement
- Valvuloplasty

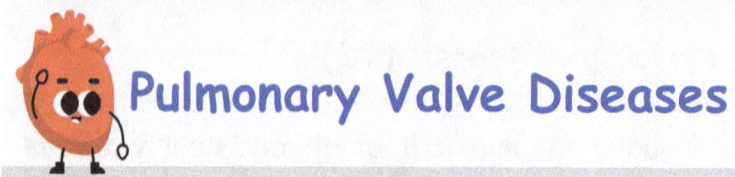
Pulmonary Valve Diseases

Pulmonary stenosis (PS)

Usually congenital and seen associated with Tetralogy of Fallot.

Clinical features
Characterized by the presence of an ejection systolic murmur in the pulmonary area, which radiates toward the left shoulder. This murmur is usually associated with a thrill.

Management
Mild cases usually do not require any treatment.
For severe cases, balloon valvuloplasty or surgical valvulotomy can be performed.

Pulmonary regurgitation (PR)

This is a rare condition and usually associated with pulmonary artery dilatation due to pulmonary hypertension. Characterized by an early diastolic decrescendo murmur, which can be best heard at the pulmonary area.

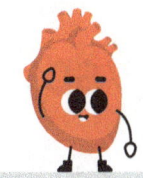

Congenital Heart Diseases

Congenital heart diseases can be broadly classified into cyanotic and acyanotic diseases.

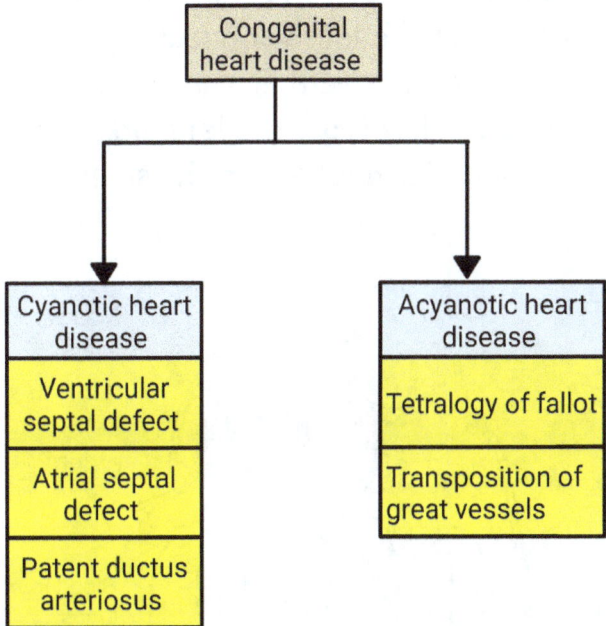

N.B:
Please note that Congenital Heart Disease (CHD) is a significant subject within pediatric cardiology, encompassing a vast and complex array of conditions. In this overview, I will highlight the most common and critical types of CHD. For further in-depth information, I recommend consulting a reputable pediatric textbook.

Ventricular septal defect (VSD)

It is the most common type of congenital heart disease. It is characterized by the presence of a defect in the interventricular septum, which results in the formation of an abnormal communication between the right and left ventricles. Since the left ventricular pressure is higher than the right ventricular pressure, the blood starts to flow from the left side to the right side, creating a left-to-right shunt.

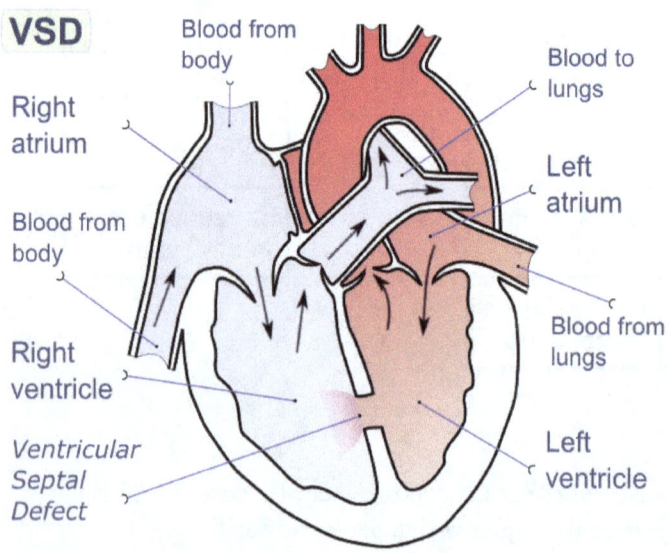

Img [2]: VSD (Img credit - Manco Capac)

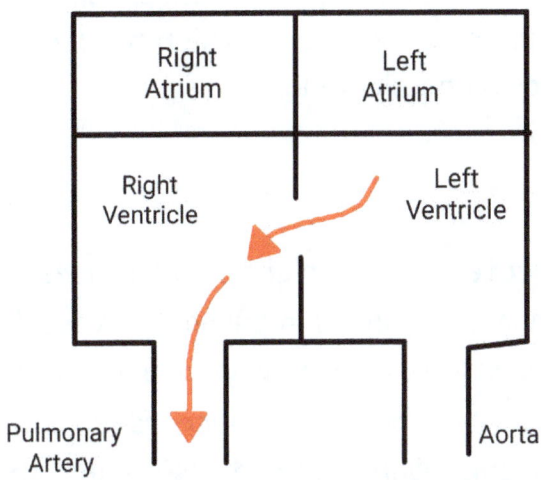

Img: Diagramatic representation of VSD

Etiology

The exact etiology of VSD is still unknown. Some cases are associated with chromosomal abnormalities (trisomy 13, 18, and 21).

Symptoms

- Symptoms depend on the severity of the defect.
- Mild cases are asymptomatic.
- Moderate to severe cases present with dyspnea, fatigue, recurrent chest infections, and heart failure.

- Untreated cases of VSD may progress into Eisenmenger syndrome, which presents as cyanosis and clubbing.

Eisenmenger syndrome

- Untreated left-to-right shunt causes permanent changes in pulmonary vasculature, which results in pulmonary hypertension. Pulmonary hypertension increases right ventricular workload and results in right ventricular hypertrophy. The hypertrophied right ventricle contracts more strongly, and right ventricular pressure exceeds left ventricular pressure, resulting in the reversal of the shunt, i.e., blood starts to flow from the right ventricle to the left ventricle (right-to-left shunt). This is called Eisenmenger syndrome.
- In Eisenmenger syndrome, due to the intermixing of oxygenated and deoxygenated blood, central cyanosis develops.
- Once Eisenmenger syndrome develops, even with surgical correction of VSD, there won't be any symptomatic improvement.

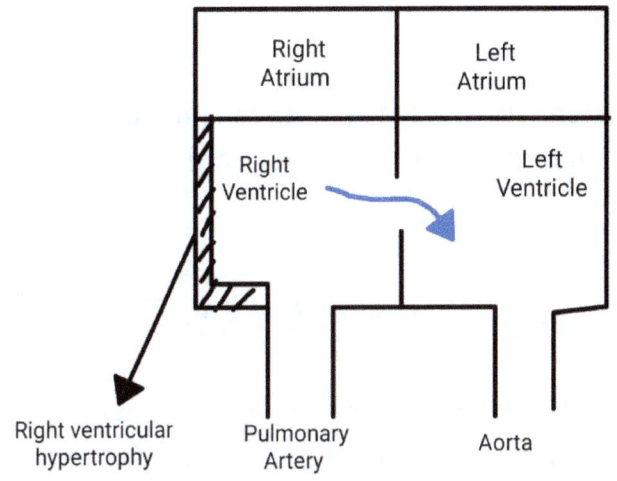

Img: Eisenmenger syndrome

*** Blue indicates deoxygenated blood

Signs

On auscultation, a pansystolic murmur can be heard, which is loudest at the Tricuspid area.

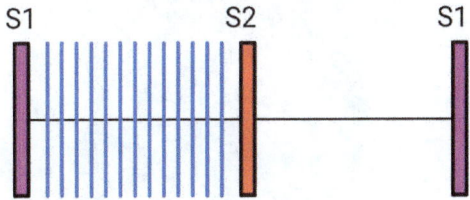

Investigations

- CXR: Cardiomegaly can be seen in severe cases of VSD.
- ECHO: Echocardiography is the investigation of choice.

Treatment

- Medical treatment of heart failure
- Surgical correction of the ventricular defect

Atrial septal defect (ASD)

It is the abnormal opening in the interatrial septum, which results in the formation of an abnormal communication between the right and left atria.

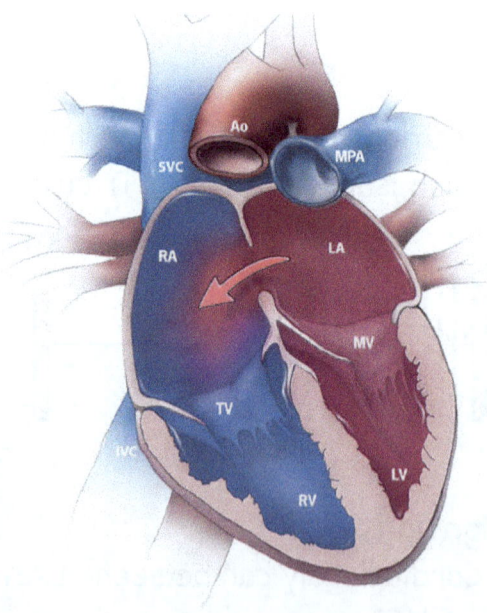

Img: ASD (Red arrow)

Since the left atrial pressure is slightly higher than the right atrial pressure, blood flows from the left atrium to the right atrium, creating a left-to-right shunt. However, the pressure gradient between the right and left atria is smaller, so shunt flow across the ASD won't produce any significant flow murmur.

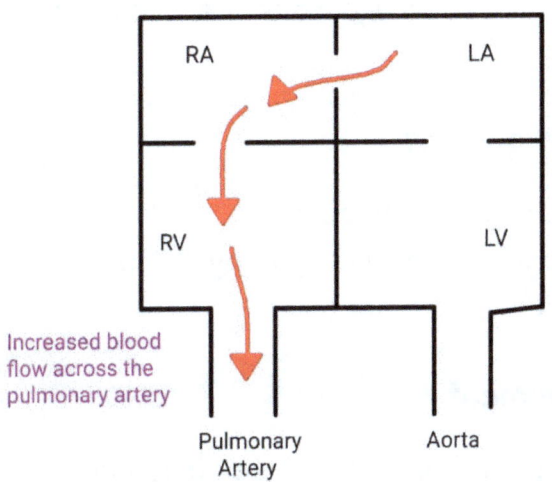

Img: Diagramatic representation of ASD

Symptoms

Atrial septal defects are often asymptomatic in childhood but may cause right heart failure and arrhythmias (especially atrial fibrillation) in later life.

Signs

- Due to a small pressure gradient, the flow of blood through ASD won't produce any flow murmur.
- A systolic murmur can be heard due to increased flow through the pulmonary valve.
- A diastolic murmur may also occur due to increased flow across the tricuspid valve.

Investigations

- CXR : Cardiomegaly
- ECHO: Echocardiography is the investigation of choice

Management

Atrial septal defect can be closed using an umbrella-shaped occluder placed through cardiac catheterization.

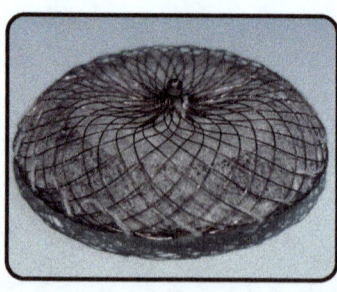

Img[3]: Occluder device used for the closure of ASD (image credit : Oleh Kushch)

Patent ductus arteriosus (PDA)

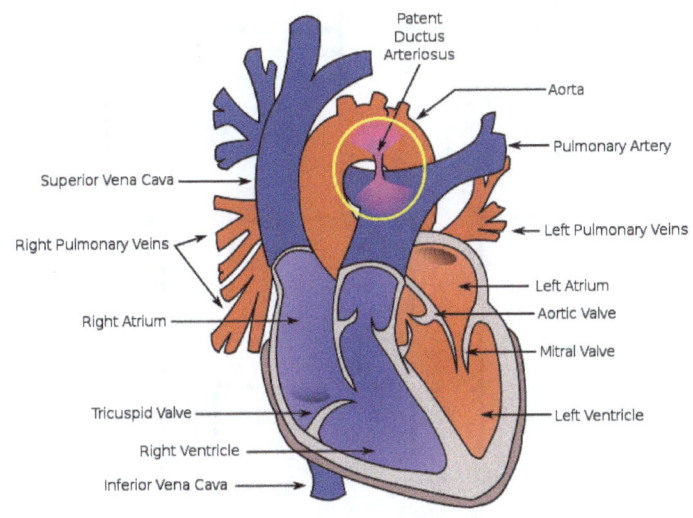

Img : Patent ductus arteriosus

It is due to the failure of the fetal ductus arteriosus to close after birth. The ductus arteriosus is a channel in fetal circulation that interconnects the aorta and pulmonary artery, and it should be completely obliterated within the first week after birth. The continued patency of the ductus arteriosus allows blood to flow from the higher pressure aorta to the lower pressure pulmonary artery, causing a left-to-right shunt.

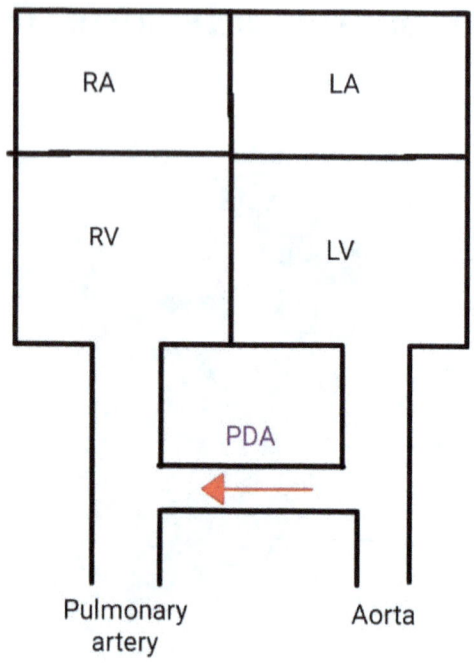

Causes

- Preterm infants : It is common in Preterm babies. But Preterm PDA well responds to treatment with NSAIDs
- Congenital rubella syndrome : PDA is common in babies with congenital rubella syndrome

Symptoms

- Small PDA is usually asymptomatic
- Large PDA presents with dyspnea, poor growth, difficulty in feeding & heart failure

Signs

A continuous murmur can be heard at the upper left sternal edge, which may radiate to the back.

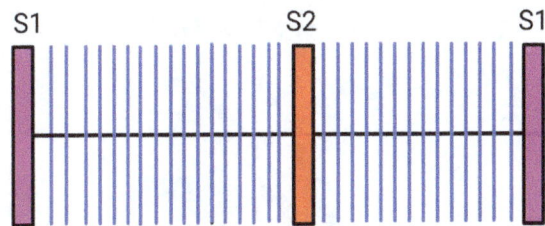

Investigations

- CXR : Cardiomegaly
- ECHO: Echocardiography is the investigation of choice

Management

- In preterm infants, PDA can be managed with NSAIDs like Indomethacin, which decreases prostaglandin levels and promotes the obliteration of PDA.
- In term infants, NSAIDs are not effective. Surgical closure is needed.

Tetralogy of Fallot (TOF)

It is the most common cardiac malformation responsible for cyanosis after 1 year of age.

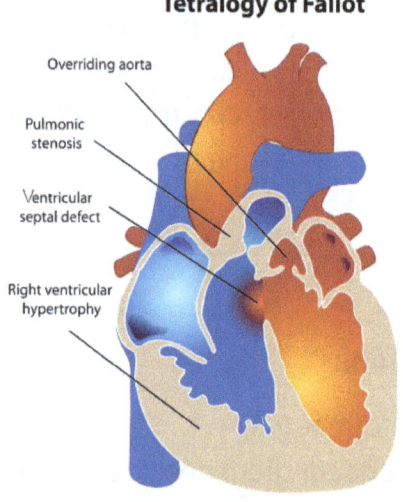

Img : Tetralogy of Fallot

It consists of 4 components:

1. Ventricular septal defect
2. Right ventricular outflow obstruction (pulmonary stenosis)
3. Overriding of the aorta
4. Right ventricular hypertrophy

Symptoms

- Appearance of cyanosis after the neonatal period
- Exertional dyspnea (In infants, it manifests as a suck-rest-suck cycle)
- Cyanotic spells / Hypoxemic spells
- Recurrent respiratory infections and growth retardation

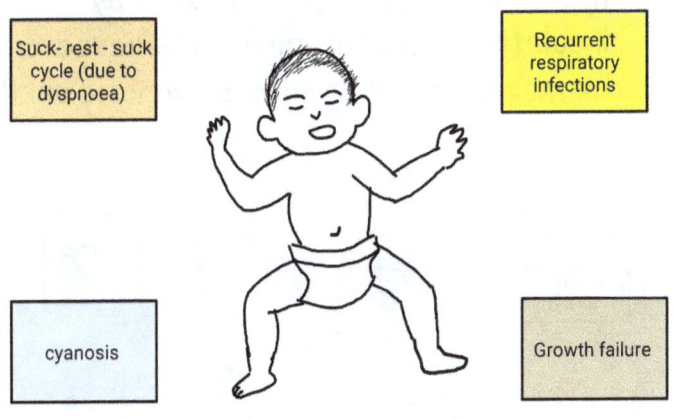

Cyanatoic spells

- Aka: Hypoxemic spells / Anoxic spells
- Cyanotic spells happen in approximately 40% of infants and young children with TOF.

- Cyanotic spells are paroxysmal episodes of deepening cyanosis, hyperpnoea, and loss of consciousness in children with tetralogy of Fallot.
- It is precipitated by exercise, crying, feeding, and defecation.
- During the episode, the child becomes blue (cyanosis), tachypneic, and gasps for breath. There may be a loss of consciousness.
- Infundibular spasm precipitated by circulating catecholamines is believed to be the mechanism that causes cyanotic spells

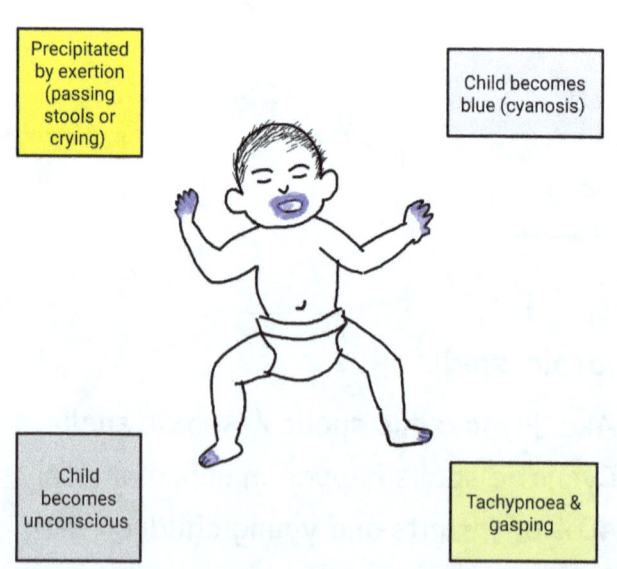

- Management of cyanotic spells:
  1. Place the patient in the knee-chest position or squatting position.
  2. Administer oxygen.
  3. Administer morphine sulfate subcutaneous injection (to sedate vasomotor centers and thereby reduce infundibular spasm).

Signs

- Cyanosis
- Clubbing
- Tachypnea
- Systolic thrill can be felt at the upper and mid-left sternal border.
- S2 is heard as a single sound without the pulmonary component (P2).
- A harsh ejection systolic murmur of pulmonary stenosis can be heard in the pulmonary area.
- A pansystolic murmur of VSD may be heard.

Investigations

- Chest X-ray: Shows a "boot-shaped" heart.

- ECG: Shows right axis deviation.
- ECHO: Echocardiography is the investigation of choice.

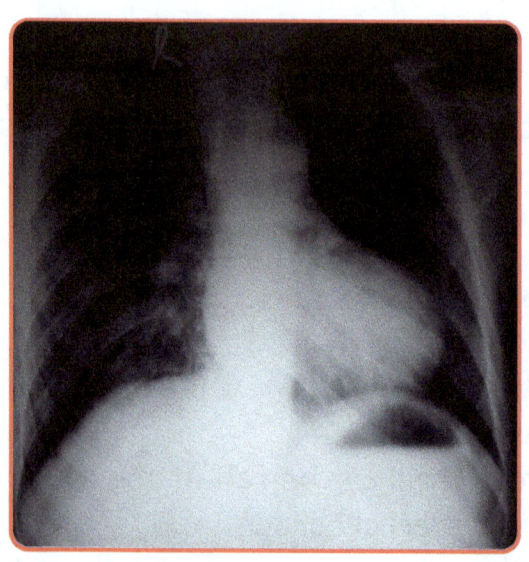

Img[4]: Boot shaped heart seen in TOF (image credit - Medicalpal CC SA 4.0)

Management of TOF

Symptomatic infants less than 3 months are treated with creating a systemic pulmonary shunt. But it is a temporary measure to provide symptomatic relief. Once the child is 4-6 months old, definitive surgery is performed, which involves repairing the pulmonary stenosis and closure of VSD.

Attribution

In this book, I have used some images that belong to the public domain and Creative Commons. I acknowledge my gratitude towards the right holders of those images. The Creative Commons Share Alike images used in this book are properly attributed below.

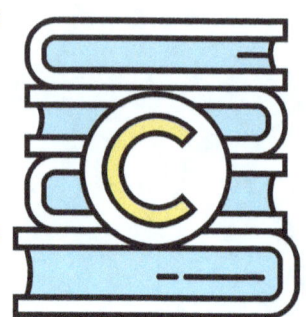

Img [1] : Adapted from the work of Theodore Dimitriou, CC - SA - 3.0 license, via wikimedia commons.

Img [2] : Work of Manco Capac, CC - SA - 3.0 license, via wikimedia commons.

Img [3] : Work of Oleh Kushch, CC - 4.0 international license, via wikimedia commons.

Img [4] : Work of Medicalpal, CC - SA - 4.0 international licence, via wikimedia commons.

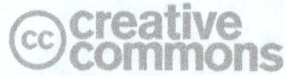

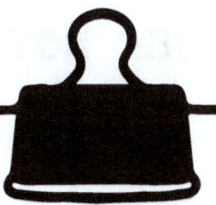

Hello future doctors and nurses!
I have put together this guide to help you grasp the concepts of heart murmurs in a straightforward and easy-to-understand manner, so you can ace your exams. I hope this quick revision guide proves to be useful for you. This is my debut book in clinical medicine, so I value your feedback. Feel free to share your thoughts and suggestions with me at sivajithpr93@gmail.com. Wishing you a fun and productive learning journey!

" HAPPY LEARNING "

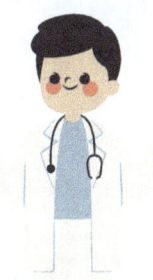

Your notes

Your notes

Your notes

Your notes

Your notes

Your notes

www.ingramcontent.com/pod-product-compliance
Lightning Source LLC
Chambersburg PA
CBHW070318230526
45470CB00002B/928